Praise for *Healing Childhood Trauma*

The usual, almost stereotypical response to trauma is to become a victim. Robin Marvel shows there is another way. We can choose to become better, stronger people as a response to bad things in our past. Suffering can be the spur to growth. I've been there myself and have led many hundreds of clients along the same path. Reading Robin's touching personal account will inspire you to choose positivity instead of self-pity and self-hatred. This little book is full of quotes like, "Life is not happening to us; it is responding to us." Put Robin's attitudes into your toolkit, and you can transform your reality.

Bob Rich, PhD, author of
From Depression to Contentment

In *Healing Childhood Trauma*, Robin Marvel uses personal, heartbreaking stories of childhood trauma to encourage those struggling with post-traumatic stress. Her focus on post-traumatic growth brings a message of hope. Robin advocates the uses of adversity and the importance of choice in bringing about empowerment. The exercises assist readers in changing their perspective on the trauma and moving them toward greater self-esteem. This guide is useful for those seeking to rediscover their self-worth and calls them to be honest with themselves and to take responsibility for their future. The author puts the power of choosing one's path squarely on the PTSD sufferer to change his/her life from victim to empowered survivor and shows him/her ways to accomplish that. This book brings an uplifting message of the ability to succeed and have joy in life, despite experiencing trauma.

Diane Wing, M.A., author of
The Happiness Perspective: Seeing Your Life Differently

Healing Childhood Trauma by Robin Marvel is a memoir of terror that evolves into a book of instruction and guidance toward self-awareness and healing. Marvel has written an easy, readable book in the field of PTSD by creating space for the reader to reflect on, respond to and learn about personal childhood trauma that creeps into adulthood in a silent stream of actions and reactions. As Marvel explains, "Trauma creates changes you do not choose; healing is about creating change you do choose." The spaces provided for inner healing journaling bring the reader into many of the needed steps to recovery. I especially liked the exercise, "Forgiveness Release" using rocks! Marvel's newest book is for anyone who experienced childhood trauma of any kind and needs to begin the journey of healing and recovery.

Barbara Sinor, Ph.D., author of
***Gifts From the Child Within* and**
Inspirational Musing: Insights Through Healing

"*Healing Childhood Trauma* is a poignant, compelling, honest book that will help you find the power to move from victim to victor, from trauma to triumph. A beautiful illustration of why you should fight to find your self-worth with practical guidance and powerful tools to take steps toward healing. A must read!

Michelle Spisz - 8th grade educator,
anthropologist and foster/adoption advocate

Author Robin Marvel hits a homerun with *Healing Childhood Trauma*. It's not just a book for reading-it's also a workbook that helps the adult survivor of childhood trauma find a new focus and develop new understanding of themselves while embarking on a healing journey.

John Patrick McCarron, Louisiana ambassador,
National Association of Adult Survivors of Child Abuse

Robin is a prime example of how victimhood can be overcome and transformed to victory. Her book contains a wealth of information and strategies, gleaned from personal experience. It will assist anyone who has suffered early trauma in life to turn it around and use those experiences to propel him/herself into a life of success and happiness. Robin knows that within each of us is a powerful force to heal, despite whatever life throws at us. And within her words, she shows us that the key to unlock that potential is self-responsibility. Robin's theme concurs with Steve Maraboli's statement, "The victim mindset dilutes the human potential. By not accepting responsibility for our circumstances, we greatly reduce our power to change them." Congratulations, Robin, for being a shining light to all.

Rinnell Kelly,
spiritual healer and vibrational medicine practitioner

"The meaning a situation has is dependent on what you decide it means." In a personal yet poignant voice, *Healing Childhood Trauma* by Robin Marvel helps us understand why some people remain defined by their childhood trauma while others define new empowered paths of healing and growth. Marvel weaves together a compassionate blend of trauma exploration and anecdotal evidence supported with self-help exercises, mapping out a process for readers to transform their pain into purpose. This little book is not light. It just may change your perspective on how you live the rest of your life.

Holli Kenley, MA, MFT, author of *Daughters Betrayed By*
Their Mothers: Moving From Brokenness To Wholeness

Robin has outdone herself once again. She writes from her own experiences of pretty severe trauma and has used that knowledge to enable others to overcome their own. As you read the book, you are constantly hit with, "WOW! She is describing ME and my feelings exactly!" She gives insight into what really helps, not just theories. Outstanding!

Ramona Clemente,
retired social worker for state of Michigan (32 years)

Healing Childhood Trauma is a hit! I really enjoyed the interactive portions - my Ace Test score is 6. It described a lot of my childhood trauma, the result of having Polio. Although I have lived dysfunctionally for a long time, I have learned a lot of tools from this book that I will use going forward. Thank you! Continue onward and upward! Girl power!

Lesa Quade, host of The Flaminpit Show, author of
Hardcore Suvivor! A Life of Heartache and Pain

Robin's *Healing Childhood Trauma* provides insights and personal growth tips that will give the reader the permission to approach trauma in a different (and positive) way. The hands-on approach with self-reflection exercises throughout this book will help move PTSD victims to champions of life. This is the go-to book on recovering from childhood trauma. Bravo!

Michael Levitt, CEO of Breakfast Leadership, author of
369 Days: How To Survive A Year of Worst-Case Scenarios

Nowadays, it is almost impossible to move through life unscathed and unscarred. Luckily, the techniques offered within these pages provide simple yet effective strategies that will enable you to become empowered, as opposed to hampered, by your past. In this gem of a book, Robin Marvel shows us how to revise our internal scripts so that we can learn to love ourselves. *Healing Childhood Trauma* is a must-read for anyone who has ever experienced trauma (which is nearly everyone). Read it, digest it, engage with it and create a life of true and lasting freedom!

Daralyse Lyons, award-winning author and journalist

In her book *Healing Childhood Trauma*, Robin Marvel has created a beautiful handbook for healing from trauma. Based on practices she built from her own life experiences, she offers straightforward exercises for readers, helping them accept their pain without judgment, as well as practical steps they can take to move above and beyond being trapped in their past.

Robin's basic message is that each of us has the power of choice: to change our self-perception, to forgive others, to be grateful, to heal and to take action. More importantly, readers will understand that there is no set timeline for healing. Each of us is unique and responds to trauma and adversity in our own personal way. For some, healing can happen quickly; for others, it may take years of repeated moments of choosing to see through a positive lens, rather than through what Robin calls "The Wounded Eye." Robin herself is a pillar of strength, wisdom and guidance that inspires all of us to take control of our lives and make the difference our world needs.

Anita Casalina, writer and director of
Imaginary Walls: A Film About Healing Racism

Robin Marvel does an excellent job of guiding those who have experienced childhood trauma into a place of healing and empowerment. She helps the reader re-identify their traumas from a victim mindset to viewing their experiences as something that they have survived from and therefore have gained strength from. With this new found power and empathy, Robin encourages her readers to continue their healing by helping others who struggle with similar traumas. Ultimately through this book, Robin serves as a beacon to help others discover their light and shine it into the darkness of their deepest wounds so they may heal and regain better control of their life again.

Erica L Spencer, Licensed Acupuncturist

Healing Childhood Trauma

Transforming Pain into Purpose
with Post-Traumatic Growth

Robin Marvel

Foreword by Bernie Siegel, M.D.

Loving Healing Press
Ann Arbor, MI

Healing Childhood Trauma: Transforming Pain into Purpose with Post-Traumatic Growth

Copyright © 2020 by Robin Marvel

978-1-61599-496-0 paperback
978-1-61599-497-7 hardcover
978-1-61599-498-4 ebook

Library of Congress Cataloging-in-Publication Data

Names: Marvel, Robin, 1979- author.
Title: Healing childhood trauma : transforming pain into purpose with
    post-traumatic growth / Robin Marvel.
Description: 1st edition. | Ann Arbor, MI : Loving Healing Press, [2020] |
    Includes bibliographical references and index. | Summary: "A layman's
    introduction to Post-Traumatic Growth and how to achieve it by
resolving
    childhood traumas through self-help exercises"-- Provided by publisher.
Identifiers: LCCN 2020007231 (print) | LCCN 2020007232 (ebook) |
ISBN
    9781615994960 (trade paperback) | ISBN 9781615994977 (hardcover) |
ISBN
    9781615994984 (adobe pdf) | ISBN 9781615994984 (kindle edition)
Subjects: LCSH: Post-traumatic stress disorder in children--Treatment. |
    Posttraumatic growth.
Classification: LCC RJ506.P55 M37 2020   (print) | LCC RJ506.P55
(ebook) |
    DDC 618.92/8521--dc23
LC record available at https://lccn.loc.gov/2020007231
LC ebook record available at https://lccn.loc.gov/2020007232

Published by
Loving Healing Press   www.LHPress.com
5145 Pontiac Trail   info@LHPress.com
Ann Arbor, MI 48105   tollfree 888-761-6268

Dedicated to my girls. You have been my greatest loves, my most valuable lessons, my greatest joys, and the reason life always makes sense. I am forever grateful to every single one of you.

Dedicated to my mom. Thank you for being a person of acceptance; no matter the situation, you have always loved me unconditionally. Your strength is something that has influenced my entire life. Thank you.

Also by Robin Marvel

Framing a Family: Building a Foundation to Raise Confident Children

Life Check: 7 Steps to Balance Your Life

Reshaping Reality: Creating Your Life

Awakening Consciousness: A Woman's Guide!

Awakening Consciousness: A Boy's Guide!

Awakening Consciousness: A Girl's Guide!

Contents

Table of Exercises

Foreword by Bernie Siegel, M.D.

Many years ago, while helping cancer patients, I learned that survivors of any kind of pain or trauma have much to teach us all. Robin Marvel's book, *Healing Childhood Trauma*, shares the wisdom of what her experience with the pain and trauma of life taught her. When we ask ourselves what the pain of our experience feels like, the words we use tell us what needs to be eliminated from life that will allow us to heal.

Also, when we find self-love and eliminate the childhood abuse that destroys our self-image, magic happens. The pain then becomes a labor pain, which leads to more than just growth-it leads to our birthing our authentic selves and the experience of the pain being worthwhile.

Have the courage to rebirth yourself and don't be afraid of the challenge. This book is not about you doing what Robin was able to do but about taking the challenge. Here is the guidebook to your becoming your authentic self—and you cannot fail. I would suggest putting up photos of yourself as a child around your home and workplace; I call them shrines, and love that child every time you see a photograph.

Bernie Siegel, MD, author of *365 Prescriptions For the Soul* and *The Art of Healing*

Introduction

It is not the burden we carry—
it is the way we carry it.

Post-traumatic stress is a reality for 60 percent of men and 50 percent of women. Although everyone experiences at least one trauma, most endure much more than that. Not only does trauma affect the person experiencing the event, but it also ripples out to the people in that individual's life, leaving a wake of pain.

Post-traumatic growth (PTG), a groundbreaking understanding developed in the mid-1990s by psychologists Richard Tedeschi and Lawrence Calhoun, can be understood and utilized in daily living to turn pain into purpose, encouraging healing instead of staying stuck in victimhood. In this book, I'll show you how to use your traumatic experiences and all the emotions involved to explore growth that will lead you to a life of strength, confidence, success, and happiness—both personally and professionally. It is time to let go of the adversity and hurt you have been carrying around.

We all suffer accidents, loss, disasters, and other adverse experiences. The idea of being able to gain positive change through such events seems to go against what we have been taught. Nevertheless, more and more people each day have chosen growth and strength versus allowing their trauma to define who they are. They are taking charge, making their lives more purposeful and meaningful, and proving that adversity can strengthen them.

Just by picking up this book, you have decided that you are ready to heal, ready to become the hero of your own story. Rest assured that you are not alone in your tribulations. I am living proof that post-traumatic growth has the power to take your life from struggle to success. As far back as I can remember, my life was peppered with abuse, addiction, homelessness, kidnappings, and many other traumatic events; later, I experienced sexual abuse and teen pregnancy. I look forward to sharing my story with you throughout the pages of this book.

Surviving trauma from childhood all the way through adulthood can leave you questioning life and feeling like damaged goods. However, when you choose to use that adversity for growth, you have the capacity to function through the trauma and create a lifetime of purpose and clarity in every aspect of our lives. It raises you to a higher level of functioning as you become ready to thrive!

Part I:
Trauma Changed It All

Discovering Self

Trauma creates changes you do not choose;
healing is about creating change you do choose.

Many things shape how we react to trauma. The day we are born marks the start of being shaped by the people and experiences surrounding us. Our younger years are pivotal, as our self-worth is formed then. Additionally, our wellbeing and coping mechanisms are molded by the experiences we build during these years.

As you will discover throughout this chapter, your self-worth is critical in every aspect of who you are right now—all the choices you have made have been influenced by how you value yourself. It encompasses every part of your life, from the people you associate with to your career, your spouse, what you buy, your vacations, right down to the clothes you wear. Your self-worth determines how you deal with trauma. It actually can make or break you.

Looking in the Mirror (Exercise 1)

Take a moment to think about how you see yourself right now. Go to your mirror, look directly into your eyes, and ask yourself, "Do I like myself?" Really focus—quiet the voices, and listen to your thoughts about what you think of yourself. Jot down on this page how you feel about yourself right now—the real you, not the label you apply to yourself such as parent, spouse, or coworker. Contemplate the *you* that exists when everything else falls away. Write your answer in the space provided on the next page.

_____

_____

_____

_____

_____

_____

The task may sound easy, but it can be daunting because we are usually our own biggest critics. Showing kindness to our friends, our family, and even strangers comes fairly easy, but when it comes to ourselves, it's nearly impossible to be completely happy with who we are, which leads to self-destruction. We hold ourselves to impossible standards and then beat ourselves up when we fall short. One way we damage our self-worth is by how we choose to speak to ourselves. The inner dialogue is powerful beyond belief—our voice is far more important than any other voice. It is the one we hear most and listen to constantly. Parents, grandparents, teachers, clergy, and others with a dominant role strongly influence our inner voice when we are young.

If during your childhood someone consistently told you how stupid you were, chances are you started telling yourself that as well, which diminished your self-worth. Such harm can continue like a cycle from one generation to the next. Whoever mistreated you was most likely mistreated the same way when growing up.

Recently in an interview with Jada Pinkett Smith, Hollywood actress Tiffany Haddish explained that when she was young her family constantly told her how stupid she was. She believed them because she trusted them, allowing their words to become part of her inner voice. She did not pursue education or hold herself to a high standard because of their words. This led to years of doubt, low self-worth, and lack of confidence. Fortunately, as she grew up she started to transform her own voice, deciding that she was not stupid just because someone else said so. This empowered her to gain confidence and start reaching for the stars, leading her to what she is now: a breakthrough comedian and actress.

Five Most Important People (Exercise 2)

Write down here the five most important people in your life right now, the people who have the most influence on you and your self-worth, whose voices impact you daily:

1._____

2._____

3._____

4._____

5._____

Of the five, where did you list yourself? Most people don't list themselves at all. We often do not consider the impact of our own inner voices. In essence, we give our power away, leaving our self-worth up to others and their opinions. But nobody knows what is best for you, except for you. Listening to what everyone else has to say about your situation can keep you in victimhood. Empowering yourself through your own voice gives you permission to heal from the trauma and start to move forward with growth. Changing self-talk is critical in moving from post-traumatic stress to post-traumatic growth.

Self-talk plays a very important role in how you interpret trauma and how you heal. If you have believed you are a victim and not worthy of the respect or kindness of others, then when you face trauma you will feel that you deserve it. Some people say, "Of course that happens to me," "Life is so terrible; I always suffer," or "I am so stupid to think I deserve good things." These statements reflect low self-worth. Believing that you are not worthy allows you to blame others and be a victim. When you are confident and have adequate self-worth, trauma will not destroy you but instead will light your fire to learn, grow, and create something good from what you have suffered through.

Inevitably, we will all face some adversity in our lives; some of us will face more than others. Our response to the trauma is directly affected by the self-worth we feel. No doubt, the amount of stress and trauma we encounter at a young age transforms the course of our lives, creating a demarcation between what happened before and what happened after. For some of us, the adversity starts in the womb and continues on until we are adults and can make the choice to stop the cycle of dysfunction.

Trapped in Trauma—Childhood Wounds

Childhood trauma must be acknowledged, accepted, and healed before you can thrive as an adult.

All negative situations we endure at a young age change us fundamentally as we grow up. Research has shown countless times that the negative and positive things that happen in our childhood impact our lives forever. The childhood environment leaves an astounding imprint on both our self-worth and also on how we process all emotions, how we bounce back, what we choose, and how we perceive everything and everyone in the world. When we are thrust into stressful situations over and over, by adolescence we interpret life in an unhealthy way. We might begin by lacking trust, feeling unstable, and fearing whatever may happen next. Our responses and coping mechanisms become muddled.

A healthy individual facing trauma is able to cope. Later, the person entering adulthood can respond to the trauma in a healthy way, which leads to post-traumatic growth. But for those in turmoil and in an aggressive environment, coping and responding to trauma can be unbearable, leading to post-traumatic stress, addiction, and, in most cases, a life filled with chaos and victimhood. We have to consciously stop being a victim and start living life fully in the present, taking responsibility for the next chapter of our lives.

My trauma started at a young age, and it had affected each area of my life from that point into my adulthood—it even influences my life now, years and years later. As a small child (aged four to five), I experienced violence, hunger, and trauma. The memories are still vivid to me now. Most kindergartners spend their time excited about school, playing with friends, enjoying their favorite cartoons—not me. I watched from the crack at my bedroom door, night after night, as my dad yelled out my mom's name and then, when she wouldn't answer, break through the front door and assault my mom and grandma, if they were both there. I would jump out of the bed, perhaps at 2 a.m., and rush to the bedroom door, clutching my Mickey Mouse blanket, hoping he couldn't get in the door and hurt my mom. Each night that he succeeded, he battered her until she didn't fight anymore, and then he came into my bedroom and took me. Although I tried to hide, it never worked.

One night that had long-lasting effects on my psyche stands out, when he took it as far as he could. I watched as he bounced my mom's face off the bathroom sink; blood was everywhere, and he just kept slamming her face into it. I knew better than to scream, because I didn't want him to hurt me—not that he ever had, but the thought was always there. I understood he was going to take me from my mom, as had always happened. While my two sisters were fast asleep in their beds, or maybe just pretending to be asleep, I hid in my closet, covered with anything I could find, clutching my Mickey Mouse blanket, when I heard the bedroom door open. That Mickey Mouse blanket was so dear to me and made me feel safe in the worst of situations. I held my breath and just prayed. At five years old, I was so scared and knew the routine, but it still did not stop me from hoping, wishing, praying he wouldn't take me. I started to feel the clothes and blankets I had piled on me get lighter and then all at once he snatched me up, and out the door we went.

I remember vividly the fright I felt, the blood-curdling screams from my mom and from me, my arm extended out toward her in an attempt that by some miracle she could save me. But she couldn't. She stood there with blood everywhere, holding her jaw to her face, crying and begging for me. Although this wasn't the first time he took me, it was the first time he had broken a bone of my mom's. He threw me in the car, and off we went to my grandma's house for supplies. Each time I was kidnapped, he had the same pattern: he'd go directly to his mom's to collect food and blankets and then sleep in the car wherever he decided. This night we ended up at a mattress-store parking lot, where we ate peanut butter sandwiches and I cried myself to sleep. Even at such a young age, I remember looking at my dad as I fell asleep and not understanding why he was doing this.

How could he hurt my mom, and why did he always take me and leave my sisters alone? I never got an answer. He always took me back—sometimes the next day, sometimes weeks later. Finally, we moved far enough away from him that he couldn't make nightly visits.

My experiences have influenced me on many levels, from the choices I make as a parent to the way I get physically ill when witnessing a confrontation. Furthermore, I will not tolerate any abuse, mental or physical, in my relationships. I took this to the extreme once when my then boyfriend was on the phone while we had been fighting and he said to his friend, "Robin is being a bitch." That was enough for me. I moved out, as I was not going to wait for him to become belligerent and possibly abuse me in a way I had witnessed as a child. (Eventually, I went back to my boyfriend.)

I am amazed at the advances in psychotherapy for children since the 1980s. When I was a kid, no one counseled me after my dad abused my mom or after my mother left the house, threatening to drive our car into a tree. I believe that's why there's so much post-traumatic stress among those who were children during the era when I was. We were never taught to heal; we were lucky to even be listened to.

In 1995, two physicians studied how childhood experiences relate to adult health. To cover a wide spectrum, they compared a group of seventeen thousand individuals, all different back-grounds, races, lifestyles. Of the group, two thirds had endured some level of adverse childhood experiences (forms of chronic, unpredictable, and stress-inducing events that go beyond the typical challenges of childhood and growing up, such as recurring domestic abuse, an alcoholic parent, and homelessness—all things I endured consistently until I was thirteen years old). The physicians' study scored Adverse Childhood Experiences (ACE): each traumatic event earned one point. Adults who scored four or more points had a substantial risk of hepatitis and chronic obstructive pulmonary diseases like emphysema and bronchitis. This test also showed that those who suffered extensively in childhood had an increased risk of smoking, attempting suicide, becoming an alcoholic, and abusing drugs. It's overwhelming to realize how much childhood events affect lifestyles and behaviors as adults.

I encourage you to take the ACE test. It can enable you to see how the adverse childhood experiences influence your health today. You can find out more about the test at https://acestoohigh.com/got-your-ace-score/. https://www.goodtherapy.org/blog/psychpedia/ace-questionnaire. For convenience, I have included the test here for you.

Take the ACE Test

While you were growing up, during your first 18 years of life:

1. Did a parent or other adult in the household often swear at you, insult you, put you down, or humiliate you or act in a way that made you afraid that you might be physically hurt? If yes, score 1 _____

2. Did a parent or other adult in the household often push, grab, slap, or throw something at you or ever hit you so hard that you had marks or were injured? If yes, score 1 _____

3. Did an adult or person at least five years older than you ever touch or fondle you or have you touch their body in a sexual way, or try to or actually have oral, anal, or vaginal sex with you? If yes, score 1 _____

4. Did you often feel that no one in your family loved you or thought you were important or special or that your family didn't look out for each other, feel close to each other, or support each other? If yes, score 1 _____

5. Did you often feel that you didn't have enough to eat, had to wear dirty clothes, and had no one to protect you or that your parents were too drunk or high to take care of you or take you to the doctor if you needed it? If yes, score 1 _____

6. Were your parents ever separated or divorced? If yes, score 1

_____

7. Was your mother or stepmother often pushed, grabbed, slapped, or had something thrown at her, or sometimes or often kicked, bitten, hit with a fist, or hit with something hard, or ever repeatedly hit over at least a few minutes or threatened with a gun or knife? If yes, score 1 _____

8. Did you live with anyone who was a problem drinker or alcoholic or who used street drugs? If yes, score 1 _____

9. Was a household member depressed or mentally ill or did a household member attempt suicide? If yes, score 1 _____

10. Did a household member go to prison? If yes, score 1

_____

Tally up your points: _____ This is your ACE Score.

The total of your ACE points indicate how traumatic your childhood was—the higher the score, the more adverse situations you faced in childhood, the greater the risk you will suffer physical and mental issues. Research indicates that if you score 4 or more, risks start getting serious. This shows that individuals really seem to suffer if they have been traumatized severely throughout childhood. After taking the test, learn about your score from the AcesTooHigh website and elsewhere. Use your score and the information on your quest for healing.

I scored 7 on the test, which is very high; according to many psychologists, I should be struggling as an adult, plagued with a long list of physical and mental health issues. But I choose resilience; I choose to be in charge of my life no matter the situations I have faced. I am not a victim to circumstance, and you do not have to be either. No one can decide how resilient you are to trauma except for you.

The test helps you to understand why some people behave the way they do and gives an answer as to why we have a culture of victimization that can lead to a high rate of poverty, violence, and dependence on the state. It is unfair for children to go through abusive and neglectful experiences, as they cannot just leave as adults can. School provides some relief—at least it did for me in my younger years. However, when I started high school, the bullying and abuse from teachers just added to the trauma by creating yet another battlefield to navigate. Each day children continue to live in this turmoil that increases post-traumatic stress, which catches up to them as adults. They react through the same emotions felt during the moments of childhood trauma. They see danger where others don't, struggle to trust others, and respond from a place of uncertainty where nothing is safe. Many will try to numb those emotions by turning to alcohol, drugs, food, and/or many other forms of addiction instead of seeking relief and answers.

Surrounding yourself with people who are good for you is absolutely life-altering. The old saying "if you lie with dogs, you will get fleas" is absolutely spot-on. With that said, we attract what we are. When you are in a place of abuse and low self-esteem, you can bet that you will be surrounded by people feeling the same way. No one who is stuck in trauma, struggling, and feeling self-pity will want to hang around a successful person. That struggling person wants someone who gives permission to stay exactly in the same place, someone who supports the poor-me attitude.

Adults choose those they are close to, but children can't always do so. It is fortunate during adolescence to have someone in your circle who exerts a positive influence that will possibly mitigate the long-term effects of early trauma.

For me, such a person was my paternal grandmother, Eva Romine. Although my dad lacked all parenting skills and was violent and abusive, his mother was the opposite. She created a safe space for my sisters and me. When visiting her house each weekend, I felt stable. I knew I would be fed, be able to sleep, and be able to be a kid, even if just for two days until my mom picked me up. Even the tiniest of things were big for me when I was at my grandma's. One of my favorite parts of being there was having a bubble bath. She would fill the tub with warm water, and I would lie there and just be. I didn't worry about someone coming in and yelling, or a fight breaking out between my mom and dad. As I stepped out of the tub, grandma would powder me, which was special. (I still search for the powder she used, and the fancy container.) I would put on clean pajamas, another luxury I wasn't used to, and enjoy the peacefulness of her home. The greatest feeling of all was that I knew what to expect.

Parents, I hope as you read this you understand your role. You are responsible for the environment your child is living in and have the power to stop or mitigate any trauma right now for your children.

Building Self-worth through Trauma

Through time I will heal the trauma I have faced, rebuilding my worth along the way.

Can we be taught to become resilient after experiencing and surviving traumatic experiences? Can we choose a different lifestyle than the one we were raised in? Can we stop being dependent on the trauma we have endured? Can we turn the post-traumatic stress we carry around with us into post-traumatic growth?

The answer to each is a definite *yes*! It will take time to heal, action to make transformation happen, and dedication to stay on course.

Self-worth is the key. You cannot build a house by just laying down a couple bricks; you have to keep adding to it. Self-worth is no different. Accepting yourself wholeheartedly and feeling confident isn't always easy. It influences every aspect of your life, however.

As you navigate life, you develop this self-worth and make the decision on how worthy you feel you are. Unfortunately we allow our self-worth to be influenced by outside circumstances and people from a very young age. We allow others to make us doubt our beauty, our strength and our overall self. It is especially challenging when you grow up with abuse, in poverty and in constant negative circumstances. These circumstances can shake your value of self, leading to a continuation of poor choices and a low self-esteem existence. The best place to start evaluating your self-worth is to examine who you really are: your pure self—the self without labels. Who would be the self standing there if everything else was stripped away?

Looking Beyond Materialism (Exercise 3)

Take a moment to think about that. If right now in this moment you lost everything materialistic, all the superficial people you surround yourself with, and your career, how would you describe yourself?

When I shed all things materialistic, all superficial relationships and all labels, I see myself as

_____

_____

_____

_____

_____

When you have high self-worth, you can feel good about yourself when all things are taken away. You are not dependent on outside circumstances to feel good about who you are. You do not need anything to tell you that you are enough or worthy. When you reach this point, everything gets better, limits are lifted, and you are able to live your very best life.

Positive self-worth leads to choices that take you on a positive path. When my oldest daughter, who was thirteen, and I were on our way home from getting groceries, we discussed dreams and future goals. She said, "Mom, I have never felt like I couldn't do something. Most of my friends aren't like that. But not me; if I want to do something or try something, I just do it." I have to admit that was a proud-mom moment for me! And I realized that I used trauma for growth, allowing me to be a positive influence on my daughter. It doesn't get better than that.

I used to believe I wasn't worth anything. After all, I believed I had nothing to offer the world. No strong females had taught me to love myself, to feel confident, or to understand that life is not a struggle. Actually, they were all struggling and suffered from low self-esteem. My choices reflected my lack. At the age of fifteen, I chose to hang around the wrong crowd, drinking heavily, partying endlessly, and failing out of high school. My low self-worth put me in negative situations that led to being sexually assaulted by a male friend. The people whom I hung out with had similarly low self-esteem.

One night as my friend was giving me a ride home, her boyfriend reached toward the backseat, trying to fondle me under my shirt. I had enough space in the car to sit back, and then he couldn't reach me. They dropped me off at my then-boyfriend's home, and I assumed it was over. I was wrong; my boyfriend was still out with his friends, and as I started to pass out I felt a man's hand over the top of my shirt. I woke up and said my boyfriend's name, as if to ask if he was the person. The man's voice responded, "Yeah. Yeah, it's me." Obviously I could tell the voice was not my boyfriend's. I started to fight him off as he continued to shove me down on the bed and start to undo my pants. I kept saying, "No, stop it," but that didn't matter. As he started to put his hand down my pants, the light flipped on, and there stood my savior, his girlfriend. She was livid and yelling at him. They stumbled down the stairs, and that was the last I saw of them that night.

When my boyfriend came home, I told him about the situation. In the following days, I told my parents and others; the decision to file charges was made. Now, we lived in a very small town of about three hundred people, and I was a junior in high school. His family, friends, and girlfriend, who stopped the assault, were now attacking, shaming, and bullying me. It was awful. As I came forward, so did five other girls claiming sexual assault and even rape; this was a pattern from this same individual. We stood united, and he was prosecuted and served his time.

Even now, seeing him around town brings me back to that night and the fear I felt. Post-traumatic stress is triggered in these situations for sure. We all have triggers that take us back to those moments of uncertainty. It matters how we react to these triggers, that is where or growth takes place.

No doubt, my decisions to be around people like that were directly affected by the way I felt about myself. In the pivotal moment, though, I stood up for myself; that allowed other victims to come forward and face the assaults they had been through. During this process, my self-worth increased because I decided to not allow outside circumstances determine how I felt about myself. I could have felt sorry for myself because I was assaulted, and, had I done so, I could even still feel the same way today—living my life with fears and limits based on past traumatic experiences. I Instead, I started exercising my power to make things happen in my life.

I live with that mindset and, in turn, passed it down to my daughter. If I wanted to try something, I did, and I am still like that. That led me to taking some risks, most of which have propelled me to the next level of my life. I don't sit around and overthink the big things—I take that swing! I now know my worth, so I am confident that taking those risks, coupled with hard work, will pay off. If they don't, that is okay because I will have learned something.

I am not a believer in failure but in growth, hence the book you are reading right now. We all choose what to believe about ourselves and how we let our perceived value affect what we do. Take a look at celebrities: they are gossiped about nonstop; some lose their way because of what others are saying about them. And then you see the celebrity who doesn't listen to that nonsense. Do you know why? That star has a high self-worth. The person realizes that no matter what other people say or do, it is ultimately up to him or her to decide what is true. That is why your self-worth is such an important part of how you cope with trauma.

Oprah Winfrey's story has been an inspiration for so many. She faced countless incidents of sexual abuse and was pregnant by age fourteen. She could have become a victim of circumstance, but instead she developed her self-worth and rose above her situation. Oprah is unlikely to be swayed by what people think about her and because of that has become a strong example of post-traumatic growth.

Self-Worth 101

Appreciate your attributes.

No one person in this world is like you. You offer unique gifts to this world. That means that you are an intricate part of humanity and one of a kind. Start acting like it. Look at your individual contributions to life and realize that the difference you are making can't be replicated by anyone else. Use the space below to list ten things you love about yourself—not the things others love, but what you value. When you find doubt creeping in, revisit this list. Hang it somewhere you can read it each day, as a reminder to believe in yourself.

Ten Things I Love About Myself (Exercise 4)

1._____

2._____

3._____

4._____

5._____

6._____

7._____

8._____

9._____

10. _____

One of the reasons we shrink from trying something new is because we are afraid of failure. Since we were young, we were taught that if we aren't number one in the race or at the top of the class, then we have failed. Public school is the worst for creating this mindset. From the very first moment you step into a classroom, you are not only pitted against the other students, you are trained that you must be the best, flawless. If you do not follow the line, if you learn slower, if you read below your level, if you are the least bit eccentric, you are made to feel like a failure. I discovered this firsthand while homeschooling my daughters—each girl had their own method of learning that worked best for them. This highlights the fact that there is not just one way, there are several ways and we are each different. Teachers praise the student who gets the best scores, listens best, or is the best whatever. Unfortunately, this unwittingly teaches lower-performing children, who may be working just as hard, to feel inadequate. This isn't fair.

Think about how your school experience has shaped your self-worth. I have never been a quick learner, but have had to work for everything I do. No doubt, I have the intelligence, but excelling in the typical school environment was a challenge. It is still that way. I have to study and work for every single thing I accomplish. I am not saying that students with good grades shouldn't be acknowledged, because they work hard too. Rather, no one under any circumstances should be made to feel like a failure. Every one of us is different, and that goes for our style of learning too. Teachers could spend more time encouraging the kid working hard but not quite getting it instead of putting this person's name at the bottom of the list of posted scores. Is such a list even necessary?

To address failure and the trauma associated with it, you have to first understand that there is no such thing as failure. What would you set out to do if you were one hundred percent confident you could not fail? If you set a goal and work day in and day out for it yet fall short, that doesn't mean you failed. It means you learned what doesn't work and what to do to get you that much closer next time. You cannot fail—you can learn, and anytime you do so you are growing and progressing. You can't progress and fail at the same time. So stop doubting yourself and avoiding those risks that will move you forward. In the midst of inventing the light bulb, Thomas Edison quipped, "I have not failed. I've just found 10,000 ways that won't work."

Three Things You Considered Failures But Actually Learned From (Exercise 5)

1._____

2._____

3._____

Let those examples sink in. Now that you know failure doesn't exist, the world awaits! Think of all the people in the world who did not excel the first time they tried something, and now think of all the things we wouldn't have if they had given up. Henry Ford, for example, failed at the Detroit Automobile Company before founding what turned into the Ford Motor Company and creating the empire we now know. If he had given up because of ways that did not work then the automobile industry would not be what we know it to be today.

Return to these exercises to help strengthen your self-worth, understand that you are worthy of good things, and know that you will be unstoppable as you grow. Taking this perspective will enhance everything in your life, personally and professionally.

Transforming the Wounded Eye

*To be resilient, you have to be willing to change
your perspective on the trauma you have endured.*

Most people are resilient, able to embrace everything thrown at them, learn from it, and turn it into growth. Unfortunately, some people are so traumatized that they suffer their entire life from post-traumatic stress disorder (PTSD). According to the the Mayo Clinic, PTSD is "a mental health condition that's triggered by a terrifying event—either experiencing it or witnessing it". These people find themselves unable to move out of trauma, with every aspect of their life revolving around it. This can in turn cause problems in daily living.

Those stuck in trauma can easily develop a *wounded eye*, which is the perspective used to interpret life after a traumatic experience. When viewing life through wounds, the person becomes scared and intimidated. Extreme adversity causes our entire makeup to be altered, emotionally, mentally, and sometimes physically. People struggle daily just to control emotions or even perform normal functions. Depression and anxiety become normal. For example, a person's home may be destroyed by a natural disaster, causing outrageous damage. The result may be ongoing fear, uncertainty, and the feeling of a lack of control. This is to be expected immediately following the traumatic experience, but for some it can be a month or even years before they are able to feel safe and secure as they rebuild their homes and start to live fully again.

When these people choose to learn and grow from this natural disaster, they find themselves on the road to recovery. Many will prepare for future disasters, stocking up on supplies,

putting together an emergency kit. On the other hand, some
neighbors choose to become victims. They feel sorry for
themselves and attract negative attention—same situation,
different perspective. This clarifies how we have the power to
make the choices with what we will do with our trauma, we can
choose to learn and grow from the disaster and rebuild with
confidence, more strength and growing from the experience. Or
we can become dependent on the trauma, using it as an excuse
for all our life to stay limited and not living to our full potential.

Becoming dependent on trauma is commonplace. People
become the trauma; it is how they introduce themselves, and it is
their story. Everybody wants to understand what caused them to
be as they are. Sometimes their story garners attention and gives
permission to behave poorly. Becoming dependent on your
trauma keeps you trapped in the emotions and negativity of the
situation you faced.

This is highlighted on the A&E Network show *Intervention*
(2005–). This show is a prime example of how so many suffer
from post-traumatic stress, how they become dependent on their
trauma and allow it to control every aspect of their lives,
claiming their rights to victimhood. If you haven't seen the
program, here is a quick overview: Each episode covers a story of
a person stuck in addiction. The producers break down their lives
to show how they became addicted to the point of needing an
intervention. Every story plays out the same: Every addict has a
backstory of trauma—being molested as a child, having an
alcoholic parent, having an unexpressive parent who never said,
"I love you," or experiencing bullying, divorced parents, or
childhood violence. Each addicted person has a similar line, or
reason for addiction—"I am like this because I suffered some
form of trauma in my childhood, so to numb the pain I turned to
[drugs, alcohol, food, insert your choice of addiction here]."

I realize this show does help some watchers to beat their
addictions, but we make excuses for these people. Not only does
this show allow for addicts to justify their addiction, but also it
highlights how society lets people stay in the cycle of dysfunction

and addiction. We tell all those people in that situation that we understand; it's hard to live fully when you've suffered some sort of trauma. Sadly, this induces these individuals to be dependent on the trauma. Think of how many times you have done this for someone you know; we are all guilty of it. We have been programmed that way, taught that if someone suffers any form of adversity they have a free pass to live in addiction, self pity and with a wounded eye. We make excuses to coddle these people who need to be healed. The only way we can improve their situation is to guide them to rewrite their story with power, confidence, and a new lease on life.

Some events are so traumatic they affect everyone on a grand scale. Wars, natural disasters, school shootings and the Holocaust are just a few examples of massive trauma that affects us all in some way. I was first touched by the Holocaust in third grade when I checked out *The Diary of Anne Frank* from our library. I felt very close to Anne in many ways. Reading the book altered my life forever. I learned that suffering at this level existed and how awful it was that others participated in such horrendous behaviors. The words of Anne were forever etched in my brain as I tried to grasp the fear and hopelessness so many felt during that horrific, sickening experience. Reading this book at such a young age changed my way of thinking. For those involved, it created unnecessary hurt and long-term worry filled with *what ifs* and *how comes*. It also instilled a very strong sense of bravery, courage, family, and integrity. Recounting that people faced such trauma while choosing to see the brightness each day was inspiring, and I also understood that what I had went through was nothing, comparatively speaking. I looked at life differently, knowing that I needed to make a difference in the world for those suffering.

As an adult, I discovered *Man's Search for Meaning* by Viktor Frankl, another book dealing with the Holocaust. Despite the chills and fear of Frankl's life in concentration camps, this book also put forth choice and hope. Although Frankl suffered beyond what many of us can even imagine, he chose to use his trauma for growth and to inspire others to find significance in living. He lived alongside 1500 prisoners in a shed with space for 200, starving and longing for the comforts of home and to see the people they loved. Beaten and stripped of every shred of dignity, waiting to see which line he would end up in, straight to death or left to suffer the incomprehensible conditions of the camp. Being beaten, starved, and degraded on a daily basis would break down so many of us, causing us to give up. In spite of the overwhelming physical, mental, and emotional abuse, Viktor Frankl deepened himself on a spiritual level, choosing positivity instead of despair. Frankl talks about how prisoners would focus on the beauty of the sunset, and there were also moments of humor, unity, and self-discovery. This is most definitely a pillar of post-traumatic growth that leads to success.

In all traumatic situations, you get to interpret the situation. In Viktor Frankl's eyes, he never gave up and searched within to find peace and make the best out of the trauma he was enduring. One of the most important things to understand in life is that you are the only person in control of your mind. The officers of the concentration camps where Frankl lived held all the physical power. But they couldn't control the prisoners' perception, because we are all in control of our own thoughts and minds.

Frankl recounts memories of men walking through the huts comforting others, giving their last piece of bread. As Viktor writes in his book, "Everything can be taken from a man but one thing: the last of the human freedoms—to choose one's attitude in any given set of circumstances, to choose one's own way." What a statement that is, coming from a man who lived as a prisoner in the harshest of conditions. This is a testament to not only the strength of the human spirit but also how to respond to traumatic situations. Given what Viktor Frankl went through, not many would blame him if he pitied himself. But he didn't want to continue living through a wounded eye and limiting himself. This would have continued giving power to the terrible situation he lived through.

As he says in *Man's Search For Meaning*, "The way in which a man accepts his fate and all the suffering it entails, the way in which he takes up his cross, gives him ample opportunity—even under the most difficult circumstances—to add a deeper meaning to his life." Victor Frankl is an absolute marvel who is a beaming example of how we can grow and use trauma in our lives as lessons that can encourage a new way of life He used the trauma as motivation to propel himself into a life that helps others. After liberation of his Nazi camp and writing his book, he chose to grow, heal, and be an inspiration to others for another forty-two years as a professor of neurology and psychiatry at the University of Vienna. Frankl published several books and lectured around the world before passing away in 1997. This man's actions are the definition of post-traumatic growth. I would have loved to meet him, and can only imagine the energy of this remarkable man.

When you experience the stories of people who have suffered extreme circumstances and still lived positive full lives, take it as a wakeup call to reevaluate your life. Realize how you are using certain events in your life as a crutch to stay stuck in a miserable pattern. Aren't you ready to live without the pain of events that have passed?

It is time to clear our wounded eye, recover from trauma, rebuild our life, shift our views and live in a new world. This is one where post-traumatic stress is shifted to post-traumatic growth, allowing us to be free with strength, confidence and without hurt. With that being said, we have the choice to use the pain we have endured as a lesson.

Ways To Clear Your Wounded eye

1. *Choose your attitude*. You have a superpower: You may not be aware of this power you hold, but once you start using it, you will see life change all around you. You have the ability and right to choose your attitude, no matter the situation you face. Every trauma you live through can be an opportunity to learn, to

grow and to prevail, or you can let the adversity turn you into a victim, keeping you stuck and limited in your daily living. You can be thrown into the gullies of life, but instead you can choose to have a good attitude, see the positive and create a different situation. Fact: I believe life is 10 percent what happens to you and 90 percent your attitude about it. Choosing your attitude can make or break you. Ruby Bridges, the first African American to attend an all-white public school, showed us how, even in the face of adversity, we can choose our attitude and in turn grow and learn. Although Bridges was spat on and called names and some white parents even pulled their children out of the school, she seized her opportunity. Her attitude determined the experience and allowed her to stand tall and leave a legacy for those who followed. According to her Wikipedia page, United States Deputy Marshal Charles Burks later recalled, "She showed a lot of courage. She never cried. She didn't whimper. She just marched along like a little soldier, and we're all very, very proud of her." This was a huge testament to her character and set a high bar for everyone else.

2. *Reclaim control.* It's always easy to blame others when something in your life is not how you would like it to be. How many years have you been blaming others for the traumatic situations you have faced? Parents really get put through the wringer a lot of times when people are looking for someone to blame. Most parents have done the absolute best that they could—they may have been coming from a place of trauma themselves. Take that into consideration when you are challenging or blaming your own parents. Life is not *happening* to us; it is *responding* to us. Look at what has been controlling your life, and see how you can take back the control. Let your defenses down, and release the need to blame. Remind yourself that your life belongs to you.

3. *Trade out bad habits for good habits.* Over the years, we all develop some bad habits, such as substance abuse, lack of trust in others, and, the most prevalent, being negative. We use these as crutches so that we do not have to deal with the trauma.

When you catch yourself in a bad habit, take note. Make a list of the bad habits, and in the column next to them list a good habit you can substitute. Return to this list before you partake in any habits that do not positively affect your life.

Using these tools will help to heal the wounded eye and allow you to take control and responsibility for your life. It will allow healing and progression in all areas. When you take a hands on approach to trauma you are able to reinvest in yourself with positive habits and mindset that will lead you towards a life filled with happiness and more success, personally and professionally.

Substituting Bad Habits for Good Habits (Exercise 6)

Bad Habit	Good Habit you can Substitute

Part II:
Ripple Effect of Trauma

Stopping the Generational Cycle of Dysfunction

The only thing you can control is your response to the things happening around you.

Big events like loss, disasters, and accidents, have long-lasting generational effects that lead to a cycle of dysfunction, continued trauma and repeated behaviors for many generations. In some cases, the trauma cycles are never broken and continue on.

Another impactful form of trauma comes from the people we love the most, the people we trust and spend most of our lives with: our family. With family being such a complicated hodge-podge of everything good and bad in the world, it really makes sense that most situations of post-traumatic stress come from within our own four walls. Our relatives show us the way, create our early beliefs, and bring us the most joy and also the most hurt. If your parents are divorced, did you feel betrayed? Do you feel not good enough because your parents didn't say you did a good job? Did you feel neglected and abandoned when no one was there on the weekend, or you were made to feel unsafe, like a burden, or just plain unwanted? These are just a few examples of moments that can have a long-lasting imprint on you.

In my opinion, this family trauma we endure is the most painful, the most limiting and holds the most power. The members of our family are the first people we trust, the people we feel most deeply connected to and unfortunately those same people become the ones who cause trauma, insecurities and pain. Our immediate family is a guidepost to what relationships are supposed to be. The way your family functions sets you up for all relationships in your life, and behaviors pass down to every generation. If you grew up with abuse, studies show that you have a high chance of being an abuser yourself. It doesn't mean you have to become that way; you can stop the cycle. You absolutely have a choice. But it takes a lot of willpower and dedication to be the one who stops the cycle of dysfunction. Using post-traumatic growth tools can stop that cycle that has been going on for years and change everything for the family you are building.

Ways to Stop the Generational Cycle of Dysfunction

Make the decision. The most pivotal step in stopping the dysfunction is to decide that you no longer want to participate in the family trauma. Making the decision holds all the power. Even though you are probably thinking, "Well, obviously I want to heal this pain, I am reading your book after all." Making that decision can be challenging, it is a big change and will unsettle your life in many ways, all for the better but sometimes it will not feel that way. We are all creatures of habit, we like routine, we like knowing. When we have been living a certain way for a long time, it is easier to continue that way. Breaking the routine can be daunting. It is not uncommon to question if you are worth the change. The idea is great in theory and it will better your life, but with great change comes uncertainty and most definitely chaos. Look at your life and the trauma you had handed down to you, and ask yourself how stopping this cycle of family dysfunction will benefit your life. But you do not deserve to be trapped in your present due to something that happened in your past. The time is now and the power in your hands.

Set boundaries. You have to think about the reaction you will get from others in the family who are choosing to stay in that cycle. They will not understand, and you will hear about it. You will become a target; these members will feel threatened because they aren't ready to see you succeed and will feel left behind. Many family members and friends will disappear. It is hard for those that are not ready to progress and heal to watch someone so close to them living fully. The initial reaction will be to attack you verbally, bring up your past, and lash out at you in hurtful ways, all with the intention to make you feel like you are not worth this progress and change. Setting boundaries will be your saving grace.

You are one hundred percent in control of who is a part of your life, you decide whom you let in, who stays and who goes. If someone is not a positive influence, then it is time for that person to move along. I am not saying you should cut them out of your life completely, unless you feel that needs to be done. When I say, "set boundaries," I mean, for example, that when your sister calls you to gossip, explain to her that you love her but you do not have time to waste gossiping. When your parents or in-laws come over and make rude remarks to instill doubt, tell them that you love them, but you are not participating in the negativity. I am very picky about whom I let into my daily life. I have no time for negativity or rude people, whether they are family, friends or strangers. This doesn't mean I love those I keep away any less than those I retain: it just means I love myself enough to not allow anyone to bring a circus into my life.

A wise person once said, "You will continue to suffer if you have an emotional reaction to everything that is said to you. True power is sitting back and observing things with logic. True power is restraint. If words can control you, that means everyone else can control you. Breathe and allow things to pass." Read that again. That's absolute truth!

Family members have attacked me many times throughout my journey, even to this day. I realize they lash out at me because it is hard to watch me, who had lived in the same circumstances, succeed while they stay in turmoil as victims to their trauma. I was the one who stopped the cycle in my family and still to this day I am insulted and demeaned by certain people. Although they are good-hearted, they just cannot pull themselves out of the lifestyle they have always known. In most situations, they say mean things to make themselves feel better about who they are. I do not participate in drama, and this goes for this situation with a lot of people.

As I grew up, the drug abuse was rampant in my household, and I mean the hardcore drugs. My mom and dad were alcoholics, cocaine users, and avid marijuana users. It was absolutely nothing to come home from school at the age of five and see piles of weed and lines of coke on the table. The parties were always at our place, and everyone attending was drinking, smoking, and snorting. Pretty much all the adults in my life were abusers; that was just our lifestyle. This pattern trickled down to my sisters and most of my cousins too. Visiting my two siblings, one older and one younger, is like seeing my childhood. They struggle in every way possible; when confronted, they claim to be that way because of their horrible childhood. If it was that bad, why are they reliving it as adults?

I know breaking the cycle can be daunting but I also know we all have the capability to do it. When family members you look up to and respect live a certain way, it is very easy to follow that track. Although I have not ever been a drug abuser, at roughly age twenty-four I did get sidetracked for a little while with alcohol. I became everything I didn't like about my childhood. I was drinking every night, staying out for days, and really avoiding my responsibilities. I remember sitting in my living room, looking around at the walls and thinking, *How did I get here?* In that moment, I knew that I had to take charge of my life, or I would create the same childhood for my children. It was time to make the decision to live differently or I would continue on this path of destruction and become everything I didn't like about my childhood.

It was up to me to break the cycle, and that is exactly what I did. Choosing to turn the trauma into post-traumatic growth, I started making small changes, with larger ones to follow as I continued to grow. The first thing I had to do was learn to love myself. I used the exercise I introduced here in chapter 1— looking in the mirror and saying, *I love you* to myself and actually believing it. That can be challenging.

Go do it right now, listen to your inner voice as you look yourself in the eyes and say *I love you.* My voice was anything but supportive at first. I would come up with a thousand reasons why I didn't deserve my own love. So I knew I had to do something different. The next time, when that negative chatter started to creep in, I said, "No," out loud and to my face. Then I replaced the negative statement I was about to make with a positive one. This helped me to heal and really start loving myself with resulted in a positive outlook on life and growth.

Freedom through Forgiveness

Holding on to anger and resentment toward another is like drinking poison and expecting the person who wronged you to die.

Trauma can trigger the need to blame, be it ourselves or others. Blaming gives sense to the experience and provides us someone to be angry with. No matter how we are involved, if we are the affected party or if someone we know and love are the victim of the situation, we can become a hostage in our mind. We are eager to make sense of it and in order to do that there must be someone to blame—someone who we can be angry with. We find the need to create a scenario in our heads that puts the responsibility on anyone but us. Although in some cases a party could have done something different that would have resulted in a positive outcome, most traumatic situations do not involve fault. Misplaced blame on others or yourself can cause more issues and have lifelong effects. We blame and then create excuses, letting trauma run our lives. Smoldering anger can continue for the rest of our lives, exacerbating the trauma's effect. This makes the adversity you suffered worse and gives it more power in your daily living.

Will Smith shared some wisdom on his Instagram that I agree with: "As long as we're pointing the finger and stuck in whose fault something is, we're jammed and trapped into victim mode. When you're in victim mode, you're stuck in suffering. The road to power is taking responsibility." The longer we keep blaming others, no matter the trauma or adversity, the more life we lose.

In most cases, blame makes you believe you are right. Some-times others are responsible for the painful situation, such as when a drunk driver kills someone on the road. Sometimes legal recourse just isn't enough for the family or others affected, which is completely understandable. However, forgiving is important, not so much for the person at fault but for yourself. Forgiveness does not give the person who caused the trauma a free pass; it allows you to let go and feel a little less pain. You are not letting them off the hook or pretending the pain is not real, it is you saying, "I am no longer allowing this hurt to rule my life. Instead I want to stop giving power to the person who caused this hurt." It is freeing, and allows you to heal and grow.

Once you forgive, you can use your hurt to help others damaged by the same trauma. When we realize that challenges that once brought us to our knees were moments when our lives shifted, they become times of clarity, giving new opportunities. The fact is that these times of difficulty and challenge can weigh you down, keep you blaming others, and in a constant state of misery, or you can use them, learn from them and then turn them into growth that can transform your pain into purpose, potentially helping many.

One of the best-known stories that highlights how a person can face adversity and turn it into purpose by finding forgiveness is the story is the kidnapping of Elizabeth Smart. She was a fourteen-year-old girl who lived in Salt Lake City, Utah with her family, which included her parents, four brothers, and one sister. On June 5, 2002, she was abducted from her home and abused for nine months by heinous individuals. Fortunately, she was rescued thanks to the national attention her story received, including an episode on *America's Most Wanted* the following year. She was spotted only eighteen miles from her home with her captors. Once rescued and returned to her family, Smart did not let her abduction define her. She is a prime example of one who has chosen post-traumatic growth over victimhood. After testifying against the disgusting kidnappers, she appeared before Congress in the support of sexual-predator legislation, rallying for the AMBER Alert system.

Smart also started the Elizabeth Smart Foundation, which works toward ending victimization through prevention, recovery, and advocacy. She has continued advocating, all because of her decision to not be a victim but instead a victor. Although she was raped, tortured and her self-worth depleted, she chooses recovery and then one-ups that to use her trauma not only for personal growth but also to help in the healing of society. She is a prime example of how we can overcome the worst of conditions and use them as a lesson, as a tool to both propel our lives and aid in empowerment of others, inspiring and encouraging others in a big way. This is just a small account of all she has accomplished since her trauma. Elizabeth Smart continues progress forward and help so many. You can learn more about her foundation at www.elizabethsmartfoundation.org.

Many nonprofit organizations exist because the founder used trauma to make the world a better place. The pattern is simple— relating to others who have faced the same trauma and then using all their resources to improve the issue that caused the trauma. These organizations make life better for so many. You hear stories of people finding themselves through these groups and overcoming the trauma that kept them trapped for so long. People often feel helpless in the face of adversity, but when they help others facing pain they can in some ways heal themselves. The list of amazing non-profit organizations with a cause is endless. It allows affected individuals hurt by trauma to have some sense of togetherness, which eases pain, and most importantly allows them to feel active in the good fight.

Every bit helps. We are all connected, and knowing we are not alone in the trauma we suffered is something that keeps us going. As humans we thrive on connection; others can tell survivors they are not broken and not alone.

Forgiveness brings us closer to healing and frees us from the pain we have been living with. In order to heal and progress through post-traumatic growth, you must forgive the pain and all those associated with it. The number-one question I am asked in interviews is if I am still angry with my parents for the childhood trauma I endured. I can one hundred percent with confidence respond that I hold no anger toward them at all. I forgive them for many reasons, including that they were only doing what they knew how to do. They did not set out to bring trauma to my life; they too were responding to years of trauma they had gone through. How can we waste one moment by being caught up in the past experiences that caused so much pain? It doesn't make sense—focusing on those moments you claim you want to forget gives them so much power now.

Forgiveness Release (Exercise 7)

I have an exercise for you to try that will really drive this point home. Today, go and collect some good-sized rocks, ideally as big as your fist. Use a sharpie to write on each rock the name of a person you will not forgive and what that person has done to you. Then put all of these rocks in a backpack or your purse, carry them around for one hour everywhere you go—even the bathroom! After the hour, set the rocks down. What do you think you will feel? You will likely experience physical and mental relief, knowing you no longer are carrying around the burdens.

This is exactly how forgiveness works. The people who have caused you trauma do not care how you feel; if they did, they wouldn't have acted against you in the first place, so why the hell would you let them have that space in your life? They do not deserve to be a constant in your life now, family or not. Forgiveness is purely for you and it is only about you—remember that. If you forgive, you are not saying what the other person did is okay; you are saying that you are ready to own your life and have all the power in the situation. You are freeing yourself.

Take Your Power Back (Exercise 8)

Make a list now of the people and situations you refuse to forgive. Include your reason you could never forgive them.

Person:_____

What the person did:_____

_____

_____

Why I will not forgive him or her:_____

_____

_____

_____

How my lack of forgiveness is damaging me:_____

_____

_____

_____

Ask yourself why these situations and people deserve to have this level of control over you. The answer is they do not; you are allowing them to. Make the decision to forgive, for yourself. Watch how your life gets better just from this action. Repeat this exercise for each person you cannot forgive.

Part III:
Choosing Growth through Adversity

A New Perspective

Do not allow the pain you endured to be in vain;
be transformed by it into a greater person.

Post-traumatic growth begins the moment you start to transform from the trauma you have experienced. When people face extreme trauma, like a cancer diagnosis, and choose to be transformed positively, they often express how their life has changed, emotionally and, in some cases, physically. They no longer sweat the small stuff but instead get excited about life and all it has to offer. It's a newfound look at the deeper level of life, the things that really matter and the excitement of actually living. Its feelings of an awakening, a *life check*. There are three main areas of growth when individuals start to heal with post-traumatic growth. That doesn't mean there aren't other areas of growth, but that these are the main areas people report.

The first area is a change in self-perception, which relates directly to self-worth, discussed earlier. How we perceive ourselves defines us. As you know from a prior chapter, this self-perception is influenced by our parents, friends, and roles in the family and in society. Trauma forces us to examine ourselves closely, to question what we have taken for granted. For years, possibly decades, life has been running smoothly and we see ourselves confidently and making good choices. We have no reason to question anything or to look at where we are and who we are being. Then *bam*...we are faced with a diagnosis, are in an accident, or lose someone we love deeply, a relationship dissolves, and these traumatic events change everything, especially how we see ourselves.

At first, we may question our strength as we wonder how we will make it through the trauma. Then we find that inner strength, that confidence, to look at whatever the trauma is and discover that we have what it takes to make it. When facing a traumatic event life change, not just around us but within us as well, we start evaluating if we are strong enough to withstand the hurt. We may well find that we are far more badass than what we expected. The reason we surprise ourselves is that we are rarely in situations that stretch our limits. Thankfully, trauma doesn't come around frequently. Trauma impacts our self-perception in many ways: it can cause self doubt, insecurities, and fear. It can also impact our self-perception by showing us how strong we are.

How we feel about ourselves affects all areas of our lives. It determines what we try, what we won't do, and how we embrace and enjoy the world around us. Our perceptions of self are built from the moment we are born and sharpen consistently from that moment forward. We are labeled immediately and build who we are around that. For example if you are born rich and powerful your perception of self consists of a childhood of privilege and in many cases respect from those around you. If you are born into poverty you are instantly perceived as a life of struggle. When you grow up in either of these environments you learn to accept certain beliefs about who you are. Sometimes those beliefs stay with you and sometimes you break free from them and build an entirely different life and sometimes life shakes you awake and forces you to look at your self-perception and where you are headed next.

I was born into poverty, trauma, and struggle. I am the third of four girls whom my mom birthed. When she was pregnant with me, my oldest sister, Emily, was diagnosed with lung cancer at three years old. In 1978, the medical field was not as advanced as now, and my mom was told that her beautiful daughter was not going to make it. The medical professionals advised my mom that she would not carry me to full term and encouraged her to abort me. They explained that a fetus experiences the emotions of the mother and that such stress meant I probably wouldn't survive. Thankfully, my mother did not take their advice and chose to carry me. My sister passed in November, and I was born at the end of January.

At my birth, my mom was still grieving, so I came into struggle, chaos, and sadness. I grew up with the perception that life is a struggle, things are meant to be hard, and life happens to you. I followed this mindset until I was twenty-three, when I discovered I had choice.

See, self-perception is something that you can change. As a matter of fact, it is something that constantly changes, and drastically so when you face personal growth. How much of your self-perception is fueled by the opinion of others? For most people we depend on the validation from everyone in our life to feel good about who we are. When we don't live up to their expectations, we punish ourselves and feel shame and guilt. We lose our authenticity on a mission to prove something to other people.

Why? How dare we allow the opinions of other people decide how we perceive ourselves? That is so unfair to do to yourself. Other people are living their lives with their perceptions, and when others attack or judge you for not living up to their expectations, it is merely a reflection of themselves. People are intimidated by greatness and let their fear take over, so they project their own sense of failure onto someone else. Their words have no meaning, unless you believe they do. That's the thing: people can talk and talk but their words have absolutely no bearing on your life unless you say so. The power is all yours.

Trauma has a way of making us see ourselves in a different light. We are forced to really explore who we are on all levels. It's almost like when you have a failure on your path to success. You take that jump, the great risk, and it doesn't lead to that place you thought it would, so you realize you need to change your course. This causes you to reevaluate yourself and your direction. You have the choice to use this setback as a lesson, or as a reason to give up. When you decide to take it as a lesson of what doesn't work, you can apply that lesson toward your next step you redefine yourself. That's powerful, so you will find yourself excited and your passion is ignited again. Same thing happens to your self-perception when you face trauma and choose to use it as a guide, and for growth.

When you first face a catastrophic event, it is easy to let the wounds and trauma define who you are for a while. It is so easy to lose yourself in what has happened instead of choosing who you are right now.

When I was fifteen, I was a girl with low self-esteem, searching for any form of attention I could get. My self-perception was sad. I had seen myself as worthless, not good enough and just a victim of circumstance. You can imagine my excitement when I started hanging out with a party crowd. I felt acceptance, but the reality is that these people weren't my friends—they were my drinking buddies. But they showed me the attention I craved. So I put myself in negative situations that led to the sexual assault and subsequent prosecution of my friend's boyfriend I described earlier.

I continued on my path of self-destruction and ended up pregnant at sixteen. This was so hard on my self-perception and the perception everyone else had of me. I couldn't believe the way I was judged and the assumptions so many were making. Parents forbade their daughters from being my friends, which was comical to me because their daughters were doing the same thing; I just got caught.

At the moment I learned from the obstetrician that I was going to have a girl, I declared that we would not be a statistic. I decided to graduate and work hard, so my self-perception changed once again. I started to see myself as an example for my soon-to-be daughter. I delivered Emillie on August 20, 1996, and I started my senior year of high school on August 24th. The year was torture; people were mean, and my feelings were hurt a lot. But I believed in myself and in all I was doing for my daughter. I graduated on June 7th and raised my hands as I crossed that stage in satisfaction. That accomplishment was everything then, and I perceived myself a success, as a girl who had opportunity and strength to accomplish great things and go places. That accomplishment was everything then, and I perceived myself as a winner, a success, as a girl who was going places.

Who you choose to be now is up to you. You can face trauma, drama and disappointment, but it does not have to define you. Other people can call you names and attack you with hateful words and actions, but really none of it matters unless you accept it as your truth. The way you see yourself and speak to yourself is of utmost importance and will make or break you. The facts are that you decide who you are in this game of life and even if ten thousand people see you as great, if you do not see yourself that way, then you won't be. So stop torturing yourself by accepting opinions and perceptions of others. Shed that need for acceptance; be confident. Decide for yourself who you are and what world you want to live in, and create that!

Life Lived Now

*While you are busy sweating the small stuff,
the real stuff passes you by.*

Trauma causes transformation in many different life areas: your self-perception, as we talked about already, but also there is change in the way you live each day. When you speak to someone who has gone through great adversity, many will express how the experience has caused them to see their life in a new light. Life becomes something different and many who are experiencing post-traumatic growth find themselves. They are more aware of how fortunate they are to be alive, and gain a new understanding. A new sense of value is discovered within. They see that life can change at any moment, and tomorrow isn't guaranteed. When you look at life through that perspective, it is a blaring wakeup call. When we are going through our day-to-day life, we can get in a routine and start just going through the motions, until the trauma hits us, changing everything.

It is no surprise that we will all face trauma throughout our lives. Do you remember when life seemed magical, unlimited, and full of possibilities? Those were the days when you saw life as a big adventure that was there for your taking. Then reality hits, and we go through certain situations, and experiences start to take that zest for life away. It is as if when we start out we are this beautiful, helium filled balloon overflowing with excitement, self-confidence and happiness. We float through day to day enjoying each day, feeling confident that we are going to crush all our goals, fall in love with the perfect mate, have all the financial success and our health will be optimal. Then, one day, we are shook to our core by an experience of adversity. Maybe it isn't a big traumatic event, but all events that cause distress feel like big ones.

These situations that cause us discomfort and hurt are like needles poking into the once full balloon. Each poke we receive starts to cause us to deflate, to lose that spark. Some of us are fortunate and experience some positivity, which helps to patch up the holes in the balloon, and we start to fill back up, at least until another traumatic event. This is very similar to what happens in our daily living. You find yourself full of life and then one day you have someone say something mean to you, or you face tragedy, and in those moments you start to lose the excitement of life. This in turn causes you start going through the motions, forgetting how amazing life is. Depression and victimhood can follow. This way of living can go on for years. You get in that routine of day to day of just getting by. We all know people who, when asked how they are doing, always respond, "Oh, same old, same old, just getting by. Trying to survive paycheck to paycheck." These people are merely existing and have really forgot how lucky they are to be alive.

Next, the unexpected happens, a defining moment that will change life forever. This often comes in the form of a tragedy, a big one, a moment of trauma that will never allow life to be the same. When you are experiencing this, you find yourself knowing that things have permanently changed. The event causes you to take a good hard look at how you have been living, and leaves you with the choice of what to do next. You can choose to be a victim and keep living your life in the same routine, merely existing. This of course is the easiest thing to do. You know this place, you are comfortable in this place, it's easy. Or you can choose to heal, to grow from the trauma and live with a new appreciation for your life.

Choosing to use your trauma as a reality check can lead you back to seeing life as full of possibilities. You are able to patch up those pinholes and start filling up with a new sense of life purpose. This is actually an amazing thing to happen. We are able to reconstruct our inner selves, putting the pieces back together in a better way than ever before, allowing us to essentially build a new life. We can now take charge and go in a direction that will create a life that is fully lived. A new sense of appreciation guides us towards taking risks, expanding horizons and really living. Then you may find gratitude, even in the trauma you find yourself in a new space with a new story. This is a story you are writing that utilizes each minute for meaning.

Finding Gratitude in Trauma (Exercise 9)

1. **Make a list of ten things you are grateful for** that put a smile on your face. Simple examples are having your favorite cereal, or a beautiful plant in your living room. Note that it is impossible to be grateful and in despair at the same time. Hang this list somewhere you can see every day and refer back to it anytime that you need a reminder.

2. **Volunteer or advocate for the elimination of the cause of your trauma.** Being able to take a stand and helping others going through the same adversity you faced is empowering. Several organizations are out there for just about any cause you can think of, and if there isn't one for your cause, then start one!

You will be surprised to see how many small things have kept you limited and unhappy. It is sad that we need a major life event to jolt us into living a life with purpose, but it is also fortunate that we can gain a new sense of what really matters.

Part IV:
Growth in Action

Making the Decision

This is your life, to be lived your way.

After trauma, we put things into perspective with various coping mechanisms, although the idea that we can go through trauma and end up feeling better in life is hard to grasp. We are taught from a very young age how to be a victim, how to respond to certain situations and who we are. Our brain is similar to a computer, accepting input from everyone and everything around us. With the disruption of our life story by trauma, we can put things back in perspective with different types of coping mechanisms. The ones we choose play an integral part in our response to trauma, adversity and what method of coping we will take part in.

The attitude most important to growth is flexibility. When we face adversity, we are forced to reevaluate every single thing in our life story. Everything is shattered and we are left in the great unknown. Our identity is our story and when it is shook up, we are left in a space of "Who am I, what comes next, can I survive this?" Being flexible allows us to utilize all forms of healing and coping, keeping the window open to all possibilities. We are all different, which means not everyone is going to respond to the same ways of coping. Be flexible so you don't miss something that just might inspire your growth and allow you to move forward.

Because we find ourselves so emotionally and physically disheveled when facing pain, sometimes we allow our trauma to turn into limitation for everything we do in life. Past programming has taught us that traumatic experiences are something we cannot overcome, the destructive effects of these intense experiences are just too much, leaving us living our lives through a wounded eye, like we talked about in the previous chapter. The majority of the population looks at trauma as a tool to keep themselves limited, and an excuse to stay stuck.

When we make the decision to transform our pain into purpose with post-traumatic growth, we find ourselves using that adversity. An obvious form of coping is to make philosophical changes, which of course ripple out into daily living. We find a new understanding of what is really important and listen to our hearts a whole much more. The person who had stayed latest at work and collected the most possessions can transform into the person who knows that the real things are the people we love and the ways we spend time. No matter who you are, what your finances look like, what you have been through, one thing rings true for all of us: we all have the same twenty-four hours in a day. What we choose to do with these hours is where things change.

The accepted narrative is to work long hours, perhaps at the cost of personal happiness and even health. When you meet people, they don't normally ask you if you are happy; they ask you where you work. What do you do on the weekends? Where do you live? They are taking stock of who you are based on what you have, not what you are. So we all create this need to be the richest, the biggest, the best. I give you all a challenge. Ask the next person you talk with if they are happy. I imagine the conversation will be uncomfortable for them and for you, because as a human we are not used to our happiness being important.

Until...We find ourselves in a moment of trauma. Think of the person who unfortunately is at the wrong place at the wrong time and a bank robbery happens. They are faced with the reality this could be their last moment. That person is not in a hurry to call their boat or their expensive car to say goodbye. No, they aren't calling the office to say sorry I won't be in so please take care of my emails. Of course not, that's ludicrous to even think that would be important to someone facing death.

This is very clear when looking back on the worst attack America has ever faced. September 11, 2001 created nationwide trauma. The people directly involved in the events of September 11, 2001, showed what is really important. Recently it was the seventeenth anniversary of this horrific attack on the United States of America. I found myself tuning in to the history channel and watching a documentary called *Voices from Inside the Towers*. They played their voicemails and calls made from the World Trade Center after the first plane hit, both from those who survived and those who didn't. Every single word spoken was a message of love to their families and friends. There wasn't any worry about work or of their possessions but only the sending of love. Instead, simply the realization that in their last moments what really mattered were the people they loved. This is a sad testament to what happens in so many of our lives. We rush through life and forget our happiness and forget the importance of the people we love. Then we may get that unfortunate wakeup call that makes us face the reality of what is really important.

Realize that this is your *one* life. You have a lot to accomplish, so there is no time to sit around complaining and missing opportunities. If you want something, get up, work hard and get it! I personally run at a high speed all the time, the reason being that I do understand that life is a onetime shot and even if I live to one hundred, that still will not be enough time to get everything I want accomplished. So I work harder than most and in turn succeed more than most.

When we face that moment of trauma and are fortunate enough to come out on the other side and can embrace post-traumatic growth, we realize the real things of life. The secret here is that most people don't. Of course, you don't have to wait for trauma to start appreciating those important moments of life. We can use this time right now and enjoy the love and share that love with everyone. It's your choice to turn your adversity and trauma into something that works for you. We all hear many stories of people who have chosen to do that, and it has propelled their lives and careers while bringing great happiness to their daily living. This is post-traumatic growth at its finest: not allowing yourself to be defined by the adversity you have experienced but instead letting that trauma light a fire in you. Some, though, seemingly need the trauma to understand what's important.

It is important to take that adversity and trauma and have it work for us. We need to choose growth and personal development above letting our trauma keep us limited, and a victim. Perhaps we can see the trauma as a stepping stone toward what is coming next, bouncing back from that hurt, overcoming the trauma and taking control.

I think that we all have stories of trauma and situations that have caused fear and insecurities. The only way to move forward is to choose to not live from that place. Many celebrities have shared their stories of trauma and how they did not let those moments define them. Reading Oprah's story has been an inspiration for so many. She faced countless attacks of sexual abuse and became pregnant at fourteen. Society labeled her a victim and she could have become a victim of circumstance and another statistic. Instead she chose to rise above that hurt. She took the trauma and made it work for her. Healing and realizing that the situations she faced were not her entire life, they were things that happened to her but they are not who she is. We have to realize that hardships will happen and they are a part of us, but they do not have to rule us. Celebrity or not, growing from your trauma is the most powerful tool in your toolbox of leading a successful, happy life.

During the process of post-traumatic growth, it is undeniable that people experience a new perspective. This allows them to heal further as they realize the value of moments and life as a whole. This new perspective puts it all in order and is a philosophical shift in not only mindset and personal values but also in relationships.

Human togetherness is by far one of the best parts of our journey in life. We each connect differently with people and each person we allow into our life has their place in our journey.

Rise and Thrive

Taking responsibility for your life
puts you in the driver's seat.

If you are a trauma survivor, a crucial step is to accept responsibility for your road to recovery. If you take a moment to silence the background noise of everyday living and truly listen within, you will realize that the trauma you faced cannot be changed, no one is going to swoop in with their cape and save you from the effects of that experience, the hurt, the fear. It will only go away if you decide to have that happen. The only person who can adjust your sails is you, and the only way you are going to forge ahead toward success is accepting this fact. It is the difference between those who suffer their entire lives and those who recover. No matter the trauma and adversity, we decide who we become in that moment, and all the moments that follow. It is not up to your spouse, your parents, or anyone else.

They are not responsible for making you feel better. It has to come from within. Anything can happen to you, negative or positive, but the reality is that a situation does not determine how you feel; you assign meaning to the situation, which affects you emotionally and leads to your response. The meaning a situation has is dependent on what you decide it means. You can consider an event and determine that it has no meaning, and in turn you will have no response to it. On the other hand, if you decide that a situation means something to you, then you respond accordingly.

This could not be truer for survivors of traumatic events. Bruce Munsky shares his story of how tragedy changed his life on the website www.traumasurvivorsnetwork.org: "This is my story of losing a lot but gaining much more at the same time." Munsky was driving to return some work items to his previous employer as he embarked on a new work venture that provided more for his family. He struck a huge construction crane, and his life was instantly changed. After countless operations and suffering, he had a revelation that encouraged his healing and positive attitude. He continues:

> My ability to recover became the strongest when I started to believe again that anything is possible, even the impossible. I stopped thinking about why and how this happened to me. My appreciation of life became as strong as it was immediately after being able to comprehend what had happened to me... Thinking positively helped me to recover every time one of my injuries put me back in the operating room or made me sick.

His ability to choose responsibility for his recovery aided him immensely as he continued to endure more challenges related to his injury. It is in his story that we are reminded that our attitude is so important when we face trauma in any form. It is in sharing their stories that survivors can rebuild their lives from the trauma. How we decide we want our story to play out ultimately decides how we recover. I commend Bruce and all the survivors who share their stories on this website; stories such as his illustrate this point.

We all know and understand that our stories are constantly changing, consistent with our lives. We find ourselves writing new chapters, tearing out old pages and opening a blank page as we take on new adventures. We are each authors of our personal journeys, and we have the opportunity to decide what gets put on the pages of our story. Our story changes when we face trauma, when we receive great life-changing opportunities, when big life events happen like having a baby, a loss, a tragic event. Through all the great changes in life, one thing remains constant: you write your own story. You are and will forever be the author. When you embrace post-traumatic growth after a trauma, you are embracing a new perspective on your life story. You can fill your pages with negativity, stuck in your trauma and being a victim, or you can do the opposite. Allow yourself to live with positivity and enhance your life story with growth and self-improvement. Be ready to take action that will engage a life of positive change. You can be the hero of your own life, and in fact you should be!

It is time to take action in your life. Post-traumatic growth can only work if you are willing to shed the fear and the need to be a victim and accept that the adversity you have faced is something of value.

One of the hardest times in my life happened on August 5, 2008, which started as a normal day, filled with responsibilities and obligations that kept me busy. I don't remember anything being out of the ordinary or that I even slowed down that day. I went to my work as usual that night as a waitress at a local pizza pub. I was taking care of customers and cleaning menus when the phone rang, it was approximately 7 p.m. I remember the cook calling out that the phone was for me. It was back in the old days before cell phones, so you actually had to walk to the phone in the kitchen to talk on it. The words I heard will forever haunt me and altered my life in ways I never would have imagined. My former husband said, "Shawn's dead." Everything in that moment froze, and I replied "Yeah, right, are you kidding me?" He responded with the same words, and I couldn't catch my breath. I vaguely remember telling my coworkers my nephew had died and I had to go.

I don't remember my drive home. Once I arrived, I tried to understand this horrific event. It was extra-catastrophic for our family, because just five months prior another nephew was killed on his dirt bike. I think that is why part of me just couldn't believe that two nephews, both sixteen, died tragically. As we gathered together as a family and started to sort out what happened, the situation started to become real to me. Shawn had died of an overdose of pills and alcohol.

I think it is important to share with you a little bit about Shawn. He was the kind of kid who lit up a room when he walked into it. I met Shawn when he was just a little guy, and I babysat him all the time. Shawn was amazing, kind, and crazy, and he had big dreams. When I took him Christmas shopping, he talked all about his goals and things he loved. One of my favorite memories is when we went to the county fair with Shawn; my daughter, Emillie, who was three at the time, and another nephew. We had so much fun, and I got to see how compassionate Shawn was as he watched out for Emillie. He was concerned for her safety: as we rode roller coasters, he constantly turned around to make sure she was safe.

He taught Emillie cursive writing, created treasure hunts for her, and genuinely loved everyone in his life. For me, it wasn't just the loss of a nephew—it was the loss of someone I felt deeply connected to. Now I had to make sense of this all. I spiraled out of control and into a depression. It was like I was in this black hole I couldn't climb out of. I decided to see a psychiatrist. His advice changed my life and set my healing into motion. When we face trauma, sometimes we find ourselves obsessed with it. That is what happened to me—I was at the gravesite every single day, for hours. To me it was how I could stay connected with him. I didn't realize it was actually keeping me in the trauma. The psychiatrist explained this to me, so I started going every other day and then once a week. Now I go twice a month.

This eventually allowed me to heal. I used Shawn's death to create a nonprofit called *All for Shawn*, educating people on the abuse of prescription pills. It was many years ago and people were not really interested in the programs I offered. I actually was told that it was too sensitive of a subject back then. Now, looking at the opioid epidemic we have today, I am not implying I could have stopped the pill situation we have now, but I believe I could have educated people, which maybe would have prevented some of the trauma that is now a daily occurrence.

When some people go through trauma, they do the opposite of what I did. They work to avoid places, thoughts, things, and people that remind them of what they have gone through. They feel any reminder makes it more real, so avoidance is easier on the heart and mind. This is actually counterproductive, stopping the person from healing and letting go of the trauma. In essence, it keeps the hurt very much alive.

Whether we make the choice to avoid or face our trauma head on, it is important to deal with our emotions from traumatic events. If we choose to pretend or avoid them, we cannot find the value in the situation, therefore being unable to grow from it. This limits us in every area of our lives, and prevents us from living fully. As we make the choice to embrace our trauma and be responsible for feeling our emotions, choosing to heal and seek out what we can learn from what has happened. We can then use those lessons for personal growth and in the aid of others who are suffering. It unites us as a whole and in turn brings a universal healing to all of humanity

You and I Are in This Together

Knowing you are not alone gives you strength and confidence as you step from pain to purpose.

It is time to take a hands-on approach to post-traumatic growth. We can talk about it and research it until we are blue in the face, but only when we start using methods from this groundbreaking understanding of post-traumatic growth that are we able to make life changing adjustments to encourage our growth and improvement. Post-traumatic growth does not negate post-traumatic stress, nor does it make light of trauma. It just provides us with a new perspective, a new opportunity to learn from what we face and utilize it for personal growth and development.

As you embark on this empowering journey, it is important you remember that trauma happens to everyone. We all face unexpected and expected situations that rock our world in a bad way. We all have that in common, but how we respond to trauma is unique. Do not be hard on yourself for the way you feel or how you react. It has always been frustrating to me when I hear someone tell others how they are supposed to feel or behave when they are grieving. No one, and I mean no one, has the right to tell you how to react to your trauma. As was stated earlier in this book, we each respond to adversity in our own way. If you feel hurt, anger, or frustration, that is OK. You do not have to fit into this box society has created—you absolutely have the right to your feelings. People have been known to speak out against a mother who lost a child twenty years ago, saying, "My goodness, shouldn't you be over it by now, why are you still depressed?" Are you kidding me?

Even if you have been through the same situation, you do not have a right to tell someone how they should be reacting. The best advice for others is just be kind to one another and supportive. Give yourself permission to your feelings. I know that every year, I feel off around the time of trauma anniversaries, even though several years have elapsed. It's still very alive in my heart and affects me on an emotional level. That is OK, as my feelings are not up to anyone else.

Please listen to this and honor your feelings without feeling bad about them. You are most certainly not alone on this journey. Your family and friends can be a source of great support that want to be there for you as you grow through this trauma. But if you do not have supportive family and friends, excellent in-person support groups all over the world and online communities can fill that need.

Because trauma affects more people than just the person in pain, addressing the situation as a group might make the most sense. One of my good friends years ago shared with me the horrific post-traumatic stress her husband suffered from after coming back from the war in Afghanistan. He wouldn't sit with his back facing a door. When they went to restaurants, any loud bang, like a waiter dropping a tray, caused the immediate reaction of hitting the floor. Although her husband was the one with PTSD, they affected not only him but his wife and their children as well. For a while the family stayed indoors, in his safety zone, because that was where he could function normally. His family, though compassionate, was limited in the way it lived as a result. This is just one example of how trauma ripples out and touches everyone around us.

Final Thought

Realize that you have the opportunity to control your life and the trauma you have faced. Take action in your life that will get you where you want to be. You are not the situations that have happened to you, but who you decide to be right now. Walking around trapped in your trauma is not working for you, so why not take a new approach that includes taking responsibility for your life, stopping struggling and feeling depressed, lost, and unhappy. Embrace life from this new perspective and you will heal. The searching for something to numb your pain, the addictions you have developed like alcohol, drugs, unhealthy relationships, etc. will take a back seat because you will be genuinely happy.

Trauma is nothing to take lightly. It has serious implications on our lives and the lives of the people we interact with. No one faces adversity alone. Rather, we face the trials and tribulations with family, friends, co-workers and every single person we have contact with. It is a given that traumatic experiences change us. We don't change over time when facing something like a death, or cancer diagnosis or natural disaster, we change immediately. In the moment of the experience everything changes, everything. I love the quote I have read so many times on Facebook that says, "You never know what someone is going through in their personal lives, so just be nice." Think about when you faced trauma, in whatever form. I can confidently say that you changed in that moment. Trauma isn't fun or positive, no it is hurt, it is sadness, it is panic. In that moment our behavior instantly starts to reflect those emotions surrounding what we are experiencing. This means that anyone we have contact with is going to get us in that state of mind. This is part of the lasting effects of PTSD.

Many of those suffering from Post-traumatic Stress Disorder walk through life on eggshells. They are triggered by words, by noises, by situations that bring their trauma back to life. The level of gratitude I feel for our armed forces is immeasurable. The compassion and respect I feel for all the people who have gone through the trauma involved with wars is also immeasurable. It is easy to forget that your behavior during and after a moment of trauma will affect others, whether you mean to or not. Traumatic experiences cause our emotions to freak out, we lose our minds. That shows in aggression, violence, crying and lashing out. Do you remember the last time you were mad?

A lot of relationships suffer due to the adversity people suffer as children and young adults. This can cause confrontation and divorce in some cases. If not cleared and worked on, our wounded eye can really work against us in all areas, especially in intimate relationships. A woman or man who was abandoned as a child and has never healed from that trauma will bring that to their dating and their marriage. Abandonment at any age, especially in childhood, creates significant damage. There is lack of self-esteem, chronic feelings of insecurity and debilitating anxiety— this being just a few side effects of abandonment. When you bring these unresolved issues to your relationships, you are climbing up hill. You cannot trust your partner, which creates constant friction and hurt for both of you. This eventually causes separation and more trauma. That is why it is imperative to clear old wounds and embrace the opportunity for growth from your trauma. The same goes for how we treat our children. Most likely you were raised completely differently from the way you raise your own children.

Throughout this book I hope you learned new tools and techniques you can implement that will allow you to transform your pain into purpose through post-traumatic growth. Let this be the first day of a new, repurposed life where you are the hero who writes your own success story. I believe in you; let's see what you've got!

Healing Childhood Trauma Quiz

Anxiety, low self esteem, substance abuse, depression, a lack of confidence and many other mental and physical ailments are a result of childhood trauma you have endured. Uncovering, accepting and healing this childhood trauma will allow you to let go of the pain, releasing yourself from the guilt, shame and self destruction you have been living with.

Take the Healing Childhood Trauma Quiz below to find areas where you are blocked in your day to day life and start recovering from the childhood trauma that has kept you limited and struggling in your relationships, career and all areas of your life. You may also visit www.robinmarvel.webs.com to take the Healing Childhood Trauma Quiz online.

~ ~ ~

This quiz will aid you in discovering how to heal the wounds of childhood with action and confidence, providing you with day to day steps that create consistent change, leading to a positive, powerful life.

1. Before your 18th birthday, did your parents get divorced? Or did the adult figures in your life go through a serious or traumatic break up where you felt abandoned?

2. As a child, 17 or younger, did you live in a home where you were consistently exposed to an alcoholic, functioning or not? Or with a drug abuser? This does not have to be a parent, it can be a consistent adult figure.

3.   Do you feel that forgiveness of those that hurt you is possible? Can you forgive yourself for the choices you have made?

4.   Was there a time before you were 18 years old that you went without food, clean clothes, and electricity or necessary items for basic survival needs?

5.   Before your 18th birthday, were you verbally abused, belittled, told you were no wanted and/or called names by the adults in your life?

6.   Have you given up on your goals and dreams to be accepted by your family? Or to avoid ridicule from family members?

7.   As a child, did you ever feel alone in your family, as if no one loved you or thought you were important?

8.   Before the age of 18, Did you ever witness your mom or dad being abused by one another? Punching, grabbing, slapped, things thrown at them?

9.   Have you ever said, "This is because of the way I was raised?" OR "it is just the way it has been since I was a child" Do you create excuses or blame the experience of your childhood for the way your life is now?

10.   Do you find yourself allowing family members to mis-treat you, take advantage of you or ignore you with the excuse, "It's ok, they are family"

Visit www.robinmarvel.webs.com to take the quiz online and receive an evaluation from Robin Marvel.

About the Author

Robin Marvel is "that girl." She has survived mental, domestic, and drug abuse; homelessness; and kidnappings throughout her childhood. Becoming addicted to alcohol and partying at age fifteen resulted in a sexual assault, and later she became a teen mother at age sixteen., She decided to turn her life around for herself and her daughter and worked hard with self-respect and determination. Currently, Robin strives to be a positive role model for her five daughters. She chose to grow though the trauma and has become a sought-after motivational speaker in the field of personal development and growth.

Bibliography

Burchard, B. (2017). *High performance habits: How extraordinary people become that way.* California: Hay House.

Chopra, D. (1991). *Unconditional life: Mastering the forces that shape personal reality.* New York: Bantam Books.

Cilona, J. (2007). *The path: Life explained in 100 pages.* New York: Catalyst.

Dreher, D. (1991). *The Tao of inner peace: A guide to inner and outer peace.* New York, N.Y: HarperPerennial.

Dyer, W. (2001). *10 Secrets for Success and Inner Peace.* Carlsbad, CA :Hay House

Dyer, W. (2006). *Inspiration: your ultimate calling.* Carlsbad, CA : Hay House

Gandhi, (1957). *Ghandi: an autobiography: The Story of my experiments with truth.* Boston: Beacon Press.

Hall, K., (2010). *Aspire: Discovering your purpose through the power of words.* United States: Harper Collins Publishers.

Lambert, M. (2005). *Natural highs for body & soul: Instant energizers to banish everyday energy lows.* London: Hamlyn. (Motivation, Self-Help)

MacLean, K. J. (2006). *The vibrational universe: Harnessing the power of thought to consciously create your life.* Ann Arbor, Mi: Loving Healing Press. (motivational, self help)

Marvel, R. (2008). *Awakening consciousness: A girl's guide!"* 1. Ann Arbor, Mi: Loving Healing Press.

Noyes, R. (2007). *The seven doors.* Gardners Books. (Metaphysical, non-fiction)

Paul, A. (2000). *Girlosophy: A soul survival kit.* Crow's Nest, NSW: Allen & Unwin. (Children's Books, Self Help)

Petrinovich, T. S. (2002). *The call: Awakening the angelic human.*

[United States]: Sar'h Pub. House. (metaphysical, motivation)

Ray, V. (1991). *Choosing happiness: The art of living unconditionally.* New York, NY: HarperCollins Publishers.

Ruiz, Don Miguel (2011). *The fifth agreement: A practical self guide to self mastery.* Amber-Allen Publishing (Toltec Wisdom)

Seuss. (1990). *Oh, the places you'll go!* New York: Random House. (Children's Book)

Shane, S. (2006). *Spiritually awake in the physical world.* [United States]: Liquid Light Center. (metaphysical, motivation)

Silverstein, S. (1964). *The giving tree.* New York: Harper & Row.

Stein, D. (1987). *The woman's book of healing.* The Crossing Point: Berkeley, CA (self help)

Teresa, Mother. (2016). *A simple path.* London: Rider Books.

Tolle, E. (2005). *A new earth: Awakening to your life's purpose.* New York, N.Y.: Dutton/Penguin Group. (self-help)

Vaishali. (2006). *You are what you love.* [S.l.]: Purple Haze Press.

Vanzant, I. (2007). *Yesterday, I cried: Celebrating the lessons of living and loving.* New York: Simon & Schuster.

Wing, D. L. (2010). *The true nature of tarot.* Ann Arbor, MI.: Marvelous Spirit Press (Metaphysical, Self Help)

Wolfe, A. (2003) *In the shadow of the shaman: Connecting with self, nature & spirit.* St. Paul, MN : Llewellyn (Self Help)

Ziglar, Z (2019). Top performance: How to develop excellence in yourself and others. Grand Rapids, Mich: Revell.

Index

M

making the decision, 40
marijuana, 42
Munsky, B., 71–72

N

nonprofit organizations, 47

P

post-traumatic growth, 10, 53, 66, 73
    chidlhood wounds, 11
    defined, 3
    new perspective, 68
    Oprah Winfrey, 23
    Viktor Frankl, 32
    vs. post-traumatic stress, 77
    wounded eye, 33
post-traumatic stress, 10, 11, 13, 16,
    19, 29, 30, 33, 39, 77, 78
Post-traumatic stress
    triggers, 21
Post-traumatic Stress Disorder. *See*
    PTSD
poverty, 16, 19, 54
PTSD, 78, 79

R

regain control, 34

responsibility, 35

S

school experience, 16, 26
self-esteem, 56
self-perception, 53–57
self-worth, 7–10, 19–21
setting boundaries, 40–41
Smart, E., 46
Smith, J.P., 9
Smith, W., 45
substance abuse, 34, 42, 79

T

Tedeschi, R., 3
teenage pregnancy, 56–57
transforming pain, 46
trauma
    and blame, 45
    and self-perception, 54
    becoming dependent, 30

V

victimhood, 3, 10, 11, 30, 46, 60

W

Winfrey, O., 22–23, 68
wounded eye, 29–35

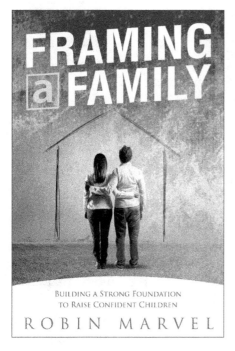

BUILDING A STRONG FOUNDATION
TO RAISE CONFIDENT CHILDREN

ROBIN MARVEL

Framing A Family will guide you to giving your children a childhood they do not need to recover from! This book will strengthen your family, inspiring you to build your home with encouragement, empowerment, forgiveness, and most important love. You will:

- Gain proven tips and tools to empower, encourage, and strengthen your family
- Let go of your expectations and embrace the hard times and the good times with an open mind
- Build your confidence as you raise the self esteem of each family member creating an unshakable unit
- Forgive, heal and move forward in the present moment with action steps that build family
- Learn tried and true methods to build a foundation, raising confident children

"Robin's wonderful stories illustrate her challenges and how she has been able to turn these challenges into personal victories and inspirational nuggets of hope for other people. I am happy to recommend this book to anyone who needs encouragement, hope, and direction to take their lives to the next level, to live life to the fullest with love, empowerment, and integrity."
—Stacey Toupin, Life and Career Coach

ISBN 978-1-61599-289-8

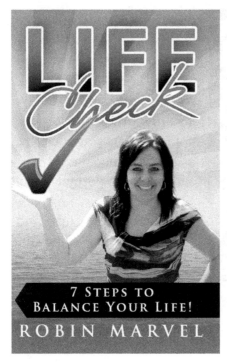

7 STEPS TO
BALANCE YOUR LIFE!

ROBIN MARVEL

About your life:

• Do you keep asking yourself, when will I be happy?

• Have you forgot what it feels like to be passionate about your life?

• Do you allow excuses to become the reason you are not going after what you desire in your life?

• Do you feel you are worth an amazing life and deserve to get all the things that you desire?

• Have you been following the crowd so long you have lost sight of the real you?

If you answered yes to any of these questions, *Life Check* is the book for you!

Life Check provides simple, effective ways to balance your life. Encouraging you to stop asking what if and start living the life you have imagined. Freeing yourself from the mundane routine of life by providing life tools that will get you rocking the boat, diving in and finding your passion for being alive!

"*Life Check* is the perfect resource for motivation, inspiration, and a reassurance that the life we are looking for is clearly within our reach."

—Victor Schueller, Professor of Positivity and Possibility

"If you are seriously ready to make the changes necessary to create the authentic life you deserve and don't quite know where to begin, I urge you to read and implement the loving guidance contained in this easy to read, straightforward book.

—Rinnell Kelly, Scents of Wellbeing

ISBN 978-1-61599-205-8

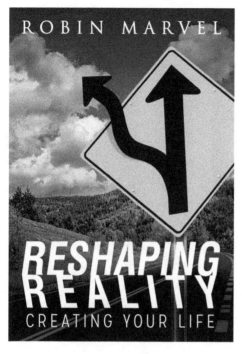

ROBIN MARVEL

RESHAPING REALITY

CREATING YOUR LIFE

We all have a story. Most of our stories have bumps and bruises that leave us at the fork in the road as to where to go next, feeling alone on the journey of life.

Reshaping Reality will encourage you to shake your spirit awake from anything that is limiting you from your potential, propelling you into a life of purpose and meaning, giving you the support needed to grow, evolve, and empower your life.

Today, you stop existing and start L-I-V-I-N-G.

Readers who follow the *Reshaping Reality* exercises will:

- Gain tools to reshape programmed beliefs
- Discover what cycles you are stuck in and ways to break them
- Learn how to break patterns of self destruction
- Explore ways to reshape your inner child
- Empower mind, body and spirit by taking an active approach to your life

"Reshaping Reality was very encouraging and spoke directly to me. It has helped me to be aware and let go of my bad habits and programming."   —Arnbjorg Finnbogadottir

ISBN 978-1-61599-111-2

CPSIA information can be obtained
at www.ICGtesting.com
Printed in the USA
BVHW041420220322
632089BV00003B/179